Women's Bodies
Women's Words

Women's Bodies
Women's Words

Wildhaven Writers

Nancy Canyon
Amy Alice
Suzanne Harris
Courtney Kendall
Rose McClean
Leslie Wharton

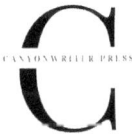

CANYONWRITER PRESS

Published 2023
Printed in the United States of America
ISBN 979-8-9886194-0-6
Library of Congress Control Number: 2023911880

CanyonWriter Press
1000 Harris #6
Bellingham, WA 98225
https://nancycanyon.com

Women's Bodies, Women's Words

Cover illustration: Nancy Canyon
Cover layout: Ron Pattern
Print layout: Suzanne Harris

Dedicated to
Ruth Bader Ginsberg

"The decision whether or not to bear a child is central to a woman's life, to her well-being and dignity. When the government controls that decision for her, she is being treated as less than a full adult human responsible for her own choices."

Table of Contents

Part 1

Telling the Story   6

Fireflies   11

Body Shaming   12

Rights Period   15

At Sixteen   16

Sorry   18

The Heart of the Protest   19

A Mother Unknown   24

"Abortion Is…"   25

WTF   26

Hold and Release   28

Chastity   29

An Abortion in Bellingham, 1972   30

Mom Held Me   32

Freedom   34

What It Means to Be Pro-Life   35

Road Rage   37

Part 2

Lipstick 40

Seventeen Bits of Bad Advice 44

Idaho 45

Natural Phenomenon 46

100 Words About Three Wrinkles 51

Dissected 52

What I Want Most In Life 53

Multitasking on Multivitamins 57

No Instructions on Motherhood 58

Take Down & Escape 60

An Endless Winter Season 62

To Me Alone 63

Honoring Your Vows 64

After It Ends 65

The Last Haircut 66

Life Drawing 68

Women Bleed 69

Set it Ablaze   70

Slow Dancing Alone in the Shower   71

Weight Loss   72

Pantoum for Happiness   74

The Gift of Self-Acceptance   75

End   79

Publication Credits   81

About the Authors   82

Acknowledgements   85

Dear Reader,

       When you read the personal essays and poems in *Women's Bodies, Women's Words*, my hope is that you will understand how we are all connected by the events we've experienced. I'm a believer in concretizing secret stories, as experiences like abortion, rape, sexual abuse, body shaming, and other covert or overt acts, seal fear and shame deep in our psyches. Telling our stories can release us from the past, empowering and freeing us to live fully.

       That said, I understand that secrets aren't the easiest thing to reveal, since our stories may be countered with disbelief. How often do we hear of a rape victim being accused of dressing provocatively? Or the sexual abuse victim asked, "What did you do to bring on his advances?" When I first shared my abuse story, one recipient said, "Oh, he wouldn't do that." The patriarchy benefits from silencing its victims. Currently, with Roe v. Wade being overturned, we feel compelled to take a stand against disempowerment and to share our stories whenever appropriate.

       The personal essays and poems in this book were penned by members of our decade-old writing group, *Wildhaven Writers*, and are the result of direct experiences. I commend my writer friends for stepping outside their comfort zones to share candidly their deepest secrets. Some members decided to use a *non de plume*, which our writing group supports. Please reflect on your own story as you read *Women's Bodies, Women's Words*, and then find the strength to share your story with someone safe.

Thank you,
Nancy Canyon, Founder of *Wildhaven Writers*

Women's Bodies
Women's Words

"You gotta resurrect the deep pain within you and give it a place to live that's not within your body. Let it live in art. Let it live in writing. Let it live in music. Let it be devoured by building brighter connections. Your body is not a coffin for pain to be buried in. Put it somewhere else."

~ Ehime Ora

Part 1

Telling the Story

When I was 16, I got pregnant the night of a '50s-themed dance. I was wearing my mom's vintage yellow dress with daisies, and my date, Mike, was wearing my dad's old letterman's sweater. That poor boy lost his virginity and became a father at the same time. We'd met at a Catholic youth retreat months before. He'd had a crush on me, told me he loved me, and then I broke his heart, rejecting him. A month later, when I saw him with another girl, I asked him to take me to this dance and, though I didn't intend to, I messed with his heart again.

In Health, we were told the odds of getting pregnant with no protection were about 30%. With math being a weakness of mine and passion a strength, those seemed like pretty good odds in favor of having sex. Yet, before our bodies even separated, I somehow knew I was pregnant. Later at Planned Parenthood, when the pregnancy test came out negative, I asked them to check again, and in a pelvic exam, they confirmed I was, indeed, pregnant.

What a mix of feelings at 16. I felt a wholeness as a woman I'd never imagined, but I was not a woman. I was scared. I told a few friends but couldn't tell my family. I'd sit at the dinner table each night, continuing to live my double life. At school, just a few months earlier, my persuasive speech was anti-abortion, no exceptions. The issue was black and white for me, and the teacher allowed me to show graphic pictures and manipulative propaganda I got from the Catholic church to prove my point. This was the same church where I'd recently been selected as "Youth of the Month" and was celebrated in the bulletin for teaching Sunday school and being a Girl Scout.

There was no one mature to turn to for advice. Confiding in friends only made things worse. No one knew at home, and confidentiality rarely exists among teenagers. At school, it didn't take long for news to spread of my pregnancy. I remember a boy I hardly knew leaning over and saying to me, "You should just get an abortion. It's like stepping on an ant." These days, I'd call that a false analogy. But at 16, I just felt misunderstood, alone, and indecisive. And, though it's irrelevant, I don't step on ants.

My friends all said Mike would want to marry me and, if he'd asked, I might have even said yes. But he was eager for me to get an abortion as quickly as possible. He hardly spoke to me, except to say he had the money. Depression pulled at me like quicksand.

One day my math teacher, Mr. Walker, kept me after class and asked what was happening. When I told him I was pregnant, he said he somehow knew. He told me about his sister being pregnant as a teenager and how this wasn't as hopeless as it seemed. Indeed, he saved me.

Looking back, I'm overwhelmed by the risks he took. Without my parents knowing, he was the one who took me to Planned Parenthood and helped me quickly explore every option, including adoption. I wanted him to tell me what to do, but he said the decision would change the rest of my life, and no one should make it but me. He did say to consider that my parents could change. His parents forgave his sister once they saw their grandchild. He said this to me reassuringly, but he also knew enough about my family to know the situation wasn't likely to be the same for me.

When I was 12, I got in a terrible fight with my dad. It must have been when I was arrested—another reckless story for another time. When I had to go before a judge, he let me go without even assigning community service. He said he could already tell my parents would punish me enough. My dad was scary during the rare times he raged. His words stuck with me. Red face, bulging veins, clenched fists. "You're so irresponsible, I bet you'll be pregnant by the time you're 16."

Within weeks, I'd found an alternative school for pregnant girls, and I'd found a place I could stay if I needed to leave my family. Andy, an older boy I knew, lived in a dorm room for priests at a different Catholic church in town. The priest let him stay there in exchange for groundskeeping, knowing he had no other home. There was a room available for me. I kept thinking this wasn't how I imagined living my senior year of high school and wondering if I'd ever be able to go to college. Most of all, how could I tell my parents? Of course, they'd know eventually. The thought filled me with shame.

At night, in bed, I'd pray for a miscarriage. When that didn't work, the next prayers became apologies and pleas for forgiveness to God and Mary for the plans I started making to kill myself. Feeling alone, weak and hopeless, I couldn't face my parents or raise a child on my own. Choosing to have this baby meant choosing a caged, demeaning life. My mom would take over the care; she'd monitor and judge my every choice as a mother. I'd suffer even more constant criticism with no escape. This wasn't the first time I'd wanted to die.

Still, I knew that killing myself meant killing us both. But if I had an abortion and killed my baby, a desperate choice, one of us could go on and, maybe someday, when I was older and married and ready, that same soul would come back to me. Maybe I'd still have the chance to love and raise this same child.

With the decision made, Mike took me to the appointment at a clinic. There were no protestors. Just a doctor's office. I remember Mike's trembling hands as he handed over the cash. It was 1982, and the cost was $350.

Doped up, it was like a pelvic exam with a sucking sound. Despite the Valium and Demerol, and despite knowing I'd made the "right" choice, I still cried through it. Afterwards, Mike dropped me off at the church dorm and I never saw him again.

I felt wobbly and drunk. Andy helped me to a single bed in a small room where I slept off the drugs. The priest offered what help he could, which I'm grateful for, but he couldn't ease the guilt, and he let me know I'd be excommunicated if anyone knew.

I woke to Andy handing me a spoon and a jarful of peanut butter. I got my things together and he drove me home, the secret still intact from my family.

Last night, at 55-years-old, almost 40 years later, Roe v. Wade was overturned. At dinner with three friends, we each told stories we'd rarely shared with anyone.

One woman had an illegal abortion in 1967. Her story sounded terrifying, but she survived. Another woman had two abortions when she was very young. The next told the story of her sister, whose baby would have had extreme birth defects. She and her husband consulted multiple doctors and their pastor before making the agonizing decision.

These are three women I've known many years, one of them more than 15, and we've never known each other's stories. It made me wonder, what if more women's stories were shared? It feels naïve to hope to eliminate the stigma of ending a pregnancy, especially a day after the Supreme Court set us back 50 years. What can stories do?

In college, still suffering from shame and the sickness of secrecy, I went to an abortion support group. After several years, it seemed incredible that I only needed to go once. After each of us told our stories, the fact that there were other women like me brought such relief.

How difficult it is, and always has been, to take charge of one's own destiny as a woman. I wonder, if our secrets became stories would our combined experiences help dissipate the shame? Would we empower women of all ages by letting them know they are not alone in ending a pregnancy for their own valid reasons? Would more men be brave enough to support women?

All I know for certain is we can't give up.

Fireflies

Remember back east, kids
caught fireflies in a jar? Trapped—
how the fireflies stopped glowing.

Like a woman
in an arranged marriage
Like a woman
fearful of leaving
an abusive relationship
Like a woman
trapped in a meaningless
job unable to afford daycare
for her children.

Remember how bad you felt?
How they too wanted freedom.
How they kept flying into the glass.
How they faded, stopped glowing.
How terrible you felt
but you didn't try hard
enough to set them free.

Body Shaming

I was twelve when my body turned against me. I started bleeding and my breasts swelled like water balloons.

At Trinity Lutheran School, in seventh grade, the teachers started clucking their tongues and shaking their heads in disapproval when they saw me. I'm sure my blouses had grown tight. They found a small stapled book on the playground with crude porno drawings and questioned me over and over trying to get me to confess to creating it. They took me into an empty room at recess and interrogated me. Out of the whole school, they thought it was me, the girl with the blossoming breasts, who'd drawn the pictures.

I started getting attention that scared me. The boys played a game where they pushed me up against the lockers at school so they could brush up against my breasts. Then they'd ask each other, "Are they falsies or real?" Some of these boys had been my playmates since kindergarten. I felt betrayed. I was so nervous walking by their table in the lunchroom as they appraised my body that I often skipped lunch.

Home wasn't much better. My two older sisters acted like I had prayed for big breasts. They taunted me and laughed about the bloody panties I tried to hide. I started spending a lot of time in my room listening to records. When Elvis sang, "Are you lonesome tonight," I felt the song in the depth of my soul. I wondered, *Why has my skipping, climbing, dancing child-body abandoned me?*

Seeking privacy, I hung out in the cemetery by our house. I was becoming a nature girl and it contained ancient towering trees. When my dad found out, he beat me with a belt. One time the welts on my legs were so bad that my mom was afraid to send me to school.

Bloomington Jr. High School was better than my parochial school and I began making friends. But even under the guise of friendship, there was body judgement and competition.

In high school, there were also greater threats when the popular boys and football jocks got cars. I was date raped in the backseat of a car. I told no one because if I had it would have been the "topic of the week" at Bloomington High School. I didn't want more attention and the dude probably would have been proud. That was my first time! Thankfully, I didn't get pregnant.

In high school I remember thinking that when I have kids and they go to high school, stuff like prom, cheerleaders, Miss America and all that sexist thinking will be a thing of the past.

Wow, was I wrong about that! When my daughter was in middle school, thirty years ago, she experienced horrid body shaming because, according to standards, she weighed too much, her feet were too wide, and she wore braces. The popular girls were mean, as always, and my daughter skipped school frequently due to the toxic social environment. She was often too sick to go to school. As a remedy, I home-schooled her for a time until she went to Running Start. The effects of her body shaming lasted into her 30s at which time she says she saved her own life by becoming an athlete.

Attitudes have gotten better in terms of sexual orientation, body differences, gender, and bullying since I was eleven or when my daughter was enduring puberty. And, thanks to people like Lizzo, there is a greater aura of acceptance around body differences. We still have no rituals or ceremonies to help young people celebrate their coming-of-age. As a society, we need more than a driver's license or church/temple occasion to welcome young people into adulthood. Perhaps a version of Bat Mitzvah but, rather than go to Hebrew lessons, some sort of community service or conservation effort would precede the ceremony. Given the backdrop of my suffering and also that of my daughter's, it is liberating to consider a ritual that would provide support and meaning during difficult times of transition.

Rights Period

Clad in her bathing suit
my niece started her period
surrounded by all the members
of our family. She was ten. Ten.
It was so unexpected.
She was overwhelmed.
Sitting by the lake we explained
when women gather together
it often brings on periods.
We sync.

A tiny dot of stone stuck to her leg.
Too young to congratulate,
I picked it off, gave it to her,
"This is your period stone."
Years later she still has that stone.

Her mother drove her to buy supplies.
Shocked on the dock we spoke
of how this could be, this child,
was it growth hormones in milk?

Imagine if a ten-year-old becomes pregnant.

What has the Supreme Court
done to ten-year-old girls,
to the parents of ten-year-old girls?

At Sixteen

At sixteen, I had sex with a boy
who became my husband of forty years.
Luckily, I could go to Planned Parenthood.
Babysitting money bought birth control
a physical exam and sex ed. I never knew
this medical care was a new opportunity.

Ashamed, I hid sexuality from my parents.
Would they have made me stop seeing him?
At Christmas Eve services, I thought about Mary.
Maybe she was ashamed too or scared.
Church taught me that sex was sin.

I was always responsible, even at six
playing house in a cardboard box
I told my slightly older neighbor
No, he could not put his penis in me
because I could get pregnant.
Mom was pregnant at the time.

Thankfully, I never needed an abortion.
If I had gotten pregnant as a teen
I would surely have had an abortion.
After marriage likely not, although
my husband never wanted children.

Twelve years without health
insurance. I paid out-of-pocket
for exams required to renew
birth control. Blood pressure check,
pap smear, breast exam once a year.
This didn't save my life but could have.

Glad to be born in the first generation
of women who have been able to choose.
Artists, professors, engineers, mothers,
children or no children. It's unfathomable
this right is being taken away.

Now, there is help with infertility,
measurements of cycles,
shopping at sperm banks,
fertilization of eggs outside of the uterus.

Society is scared of sex. Why?
Pleasure, survival of the species.
Partners should not only listen for NO
but wait for YES. Why can murder,
throat cutting, hanging, gun wounds
be witnessed on TV but not a naked
body? We all have them. Bodies.

Sorry

Once I said sorry, then sorry for saying sorry. There was nothing to be sorry about, really. It wasn't my fault. You didn't attach, that is all. Down the driveway, the day grew dark, cows grazing in the falling ash, swishing through dusty fields. No stars, just pink lightning striking cloud to cloud, like the words my husband used on us. The words weren't easy to swallow, like his cheap beer, bitter. Sorry I couldn't save you, shield you from those discounting words. I came apart the day the volcano blew. You inside me, only a joyous shadow, and then gone—a specter. We disappeared together through a cloud of dark ash. Sorry, I said. Sorry, sorry, sorry. Then you were a bright flash and I was home safe.

The Heart of the Protest

People lined the street on a cold January for an annual March for Life event, holding homemade signs with phrases such as "Abortion Kills" and "Pray to End Abortion." A mile-long main road filled with abortion protestors and many traffic lights. It took a long time for our car to crawl past them down the busy thoroughfare. I kept my eyes down, trying not to look at anyone and especially not the children chanting alongside their parents. The signs, the chanting, the fervor behind this protest sparked unease in me. Protest is a valid part of our democracy and I had no qualms with the protest. It was just that I was afraid of these people. Twenty years later and I was still afraid.

The thin pages of the telephone directory stuck together as I tried to find where the gray section with residential listings ended and the yellow pages with commercial listings began. There it was: section A. This was Idaho in 2002, and the only listing under abortion services was a small line with a Boise phone number. There were many Christian-centered pregnancy crisis centers, but just one abortion provider listed for the entire state—at least according to the Yellow Pages. We didn't have the ubiquity of smart phones or Google at our fingertips at the time, and I sure as hell wasn't going to search for abortion providers at the community college computer lab across the street.

I sat in my one-bedroom apartment with a telephone book in my lap and a scratched Nokia cell phone beside me. I punched in the number and asked to make an appointment. The deed was done.

Over a decade later Boise would have two Planned Parenthood clinics, though Idaho had only five facilities providing abortion in 2017. That same year, the Guttmacher Institute—a research and policy organization committed to advancing sexual and reproductive health rights

—found that 95% of Idaho counties had no clinics performing abortions, and 67% of Idaho's women lived in those counties. In 2002, I traveled two hours to a no-name gray building tucked in a residential Boise neighborhood to have an abortion performed.

There were no signs, and I was grateful that my boyfriend was driving and had sufficient navigation skills to find our way there. He parked in the empty lot and then it was time for me to go in. I went in alone and he drove off after telling me he'd be back in an hour or so. We were so naïve. I was eighteen, he was nineteen.

The waiting room was cramped, and over the reception desk I could see the piles of medical charts that apparently couldn't fit in any of the existing file cabinets. It was dark and dingy, but no back alley. I was the only patient in the waiting room, simply waiting until my name could be called.

As of January 2008, and up until August 2022, Idaho required that a woman seeking abortion receive state-directed counseling that included information designed to discourage her from having an abortion. She had to then wait 24 hours after that counseling before the procedure was provided. The very first sentence of the state-directed pamphlet entitled "What You Should Know About Abortion" reads that "It is the public policy of the state of Idaho to prefer live childbirth over abortion."

I, too, preferred live childbirth over abortion. Contraception—other than condoms—was not readily available, and my sexual and reproductive health knowledge was not what it should have been. As a young mother in Idaho—no doubt a single one—my job opportunities would have been in the service industry. Idaho law allowed restaurants to pay less than minimum wage because waitstaff earned tips—usually. As a waitress I worked twelve-hour days to earn $3.25 per hour and often juggled another job or two to boost my income. I survived, but I did not support another living being. The expense of the baby would have been on the state welfare system had I chosen live childbirth. Despite the state's preference, I did not choose that option.

In 2002 the doctor led me into the surgical room, as sparsely decorated and just as crowded as his waiting room. I managed to maneuver to the bed in the middle of the room and assumed the stirrup position. During this time I did not receive state-directed counseling. Nor did anyone question my decision or rationality. I made an appointment, I showed up, I was given a hospital gown. The doctor did not give me the aforementioned pamphlet. He did, however, keep the ultrasound screen faced towards me so that I could see the developing nine-week fetus.

"What You Should Know About Abortion" attempts to line out the risks women may receive from abortion: "According to data from the Centers for Disease Control and Prevention (CDC), the risk of dying from legally induced abortion is 0.6 per 100,000 abortions." A slim percentage. Compare that with the state's preference, and their choice on how to present the information: "If you choose to carry a child to full term (40 menstrual weeks, 38 weeks after fertilization) you can usually expect to experience a safe and healthy process. The risk of dying in childbirth is 6.7 in 100,000 live births." The small risk of dying from having an abortion is relayed in clinical terms. The risk of dying in childbirth is greater yet you can usually expect a safe and healthy experience. The grammatical gymnastics fascinate me.

I was not one of the 0.6, and I was not yet privy to the pamphlet or the ways in which adjectives can skew the facts. When the doctor was done, I was done. There was no counseling after, or even a moment alone to process. I was to change back into street clothes and receive my discharge orders. To be honest, I was in shock from the ultrasound and the entire process. I was numbed in a way that would follow me the next couple of weeks and into Christmas and the New Year. I didn't know what to think when I pushed open the door leading to the parking lot. And I didn't know what to make of the group of people, some with signs, protesting outside the clinic's entrance.

I couldn't understand: Why on earth were they protesting at a clinic smack dab in the middle of a residential area with absolutely no thru-traffic? To whom were they protesting? The what was clear, but the people inside could not see the protestors and clearly didn't care that they had taken up residence in their parking lot. I was not warned or escorted. I was assaulted by a well-meaning (I suppose) woman with a baseball card that she thrust into my hands. "If you need anything, honey, just call," she said. I climbed into the passenger seat of the waiting Ford Bronco and looked down at the card. As if the ultrasound hadn't been enough, here were pictures of several stages of fetal development. No phone number to call, just a finger-wagging fist to my jaw. I spent the next couple of blocks tearing the card into small pieces, tears all I could muster.

At times I wish I had kept that card, if only so that I could relook at it. In the moment, I just saw lies. I had, after all, just seen a nine-week ultrasound. I knew what a nine-week-old fetus looked like. The makers of these particular baseball cards didn't know what a nine-week-old fetus looked like, which is a generous supposition. I wish I could read it today and fact-check it with the distance that time has given me.

Three months after Roe v. Wade was overturned, in August 2022, Idaho's pamphlet continues to be accessible on the Idaho Department of Health & Welfare's website. Abortion, however, is banned with two exceptions: to save the pregnant person's life and if the pregnancy is a result of rape and/or incest. The law has been challenged due to the law's writing, which calls for health care providers to prove that an abortion met that criteria or face potential arrest. In the case of rape and/or incest, police reports must be filed, and those reports are not publicly available until the investigation is complete and a decision is reached, which can take months or even years. Pregnancy usually lasts nine months.

When most people protest, they protest because they have passion for a cause. I like to think that they think of themselves as nobly trying to right the injustices of the world. Many protesting within the anti-abortion community see this as the greatest human rights violation of their time. And that woman with her baseball card was no doubt trying to right the injustice she sees in the world. Every person I've ever seen carrying a Pro-Life/Anti-Abortion sign is no doubt trying to right an injustice.

But I cringe whenever I see them. I feel a deep heat inside my chest, and I can feel everything inside me moving closer and closer to my core. It's a gut reaction I still can't help twenty years later. It's the deer freezing at the sound of a twig snapping, with the hunter's gun trained on its heart. What I feel those protests lack is an understanding of our hearts.

A Mother Unknown

Carrying her child
in empty arms
her blank gaze
listens for its cry
as she mouths
favorite names
that still go unused.
She bore its weight
for such a short time,
wonders now why
the burden seems so heavy.
Startled in conception
frightened of its
unexpectedness—
there was no time
to argue with modern
morality. Yet
being sucked away
in a plastic tube
left her forsaken
alone beneath white lights.

She knew she could
not explain it to her boyfriend
waiting in the lobby. He had
not questioned her glazed
determination
although once they knew
he hesitated
coming to bed.
                    She
hugs close this unseen
burden like a real child
trying to hide
its face from the world
she has denied it.

"Abortion Is…"

It's hard to ignore outrage
about the stealing of bodies,
of lives, for a slogan
that costs you nothing,
until it does.

Because of course,
we all know someone,
or are someone,
whose body or life has been stolen.

Where are individual rights?
Hands off my ~~body~~ guns.

So easy for some
to condemn a decision,
cast aside
a merciful argument,
until it's you,
or your sister,
your best friend.
What then?

WTF

The baby has extreme deformation, will die in childhood.
The mother's health is at risk, life is at risk.
What about a 46-year-old mother of five, grandmother of one?
She has been taking mental health meds dangerous for the
fetus during pregnancy.
What about women that are homeless, drug addicts, anorexic, PhD
candidates, rape victims,
an 11-year-old who doesn't know better, the father is her uncle,
teenagers unaware they are late
then too scared to tell the truth,
women who have poor access to birth control,
fell under a one-night spell?
What about regret, fear, women with cancer,
women who are autistic, who cringe at the sound
of barking dogs or crying babies, who hate their husbands
but are afraid to leave, who work retail,
fast food, low wages on their feet all day,
or live with roommates who party all night,
with no family support,
Japanese women who believe the unborn are spiritual
beings but will have another chance to come to life,
Jewish women who believe life starts at the first breath and
ends at the last, or women who drink
too much, smoke too much, who are beaten by partners, or
their partners beat the already born?
What if she's had an affair with her neighbor?

What if she's in prison, had sex with a guard for cigarettes?
What if her first two children were taken away by social
service, her heart is broken?
Who has the right to her body, her life, her fetus.
The government?
What if she just doesn't want to be pregnant?
What becomes of an unwanted child?

Hold and Release

A white plastic stick with two blue lines
A man's denial screaming through the phone receiver
Another man's accusation: *You are so selfish*
A move, a run from, a run towards
Seven hundred twenty-one miles away from everyone I know
A bare mattress in the middle of a bare room
Morning nausea and self-revile
Secrets buried inside a numb heart
A Planned Parenthood, stoic and secure
A nurse's sympathetic coo: *Isn't there anyone you could call?*
A waiting room chair for one
An ultrasound image of a soul who will never be
The sound of a vacuum cutting through tears
Paper butterflies hanging above my held breath
A beige recliner, boxed apple juice, a plastic straw
A solitary tear on my hospital gown
A lonely car ride to an empty apartment
Late nights with no sleep
A book with warm colors and soothing thoughts
An image of silence
An image of peace
A breath released.

Chastity

Forgoing protests, running for office,
I design a chastity belt.
Modern plastic not steel.
The morning-after pill may not be legal
but chastity belts are. A good solution.
Women can buy them.
Husbands will buy them for unruly wives.
Parents of daughters with early periods,
who have uncles turned on by budding bodies,
parents who believe sex before marriage
is a terrible sin, can buy them.
Counselors at drug rehab centers, mental health
facilities may give them away for free. Keep the key.
DSHS will hand chastity out to parents
whose children have been taken away.
Foster care children may want to wear them to feel safe.
Women who need to think twice before falling
in love or lust can hide the key in ice—like a credit card.
Anyone can buy chastity with a credit card
on Amazon.
Available in multiple colors and sizes
a red arrow points to the clitoris
guides the lucky "let in" for sex
with a woman or a girl who lives
in one of those save-every-fetus states
to make the risk worth it.
I'll become rich. Just imagine.

An Abortion in Bellingham, 1972

I had an abortion in the 70s in Bellingham. I am so grateful to Planned Parenthood for helping me arrange it. The procedure was at six weeks and I recall only that it was in a clean, clinical setting and my interactions with the staff were impersonal and professional. It's what I would wish for any woman who decides to have an abortion.

I have no regrets about my decision, just relief. My partner and I were not ready to be parents. Among other funky things in our living situation, we were living in a cabin with a contaminated well so we had to fill up oil drums with drinking water at the gas station. We were in the experimenting stage of our life regarding drugs. The judgement centers of our brains were still developing. We were just beginning to figure out who we were and what paths we wanted to take.

Friends were dying in Vietnam, and we were just waking up to the reality of the military industrial complex, the role oil played in political decisions and how certain corporations profited from war. My partner went through immobilizing periods of depression.

I am so thankful that I did not listen to the anti-abortion propagandists (who are fine with assault rifles) and listened instead to my pragmatic, scientific, wise women friends.

I had a child years later when I was able to address the enormous responsibility with vitality and joy. I could honestly say to her, "I chose to have you and I am here for you—body, heart, and mind."

P.S. Oct.11, 2022—I drove by Planned Parenthood and there were two people standing outside with signs that said, "Pray to God to end abortion." I include the date here because I can't believe this kind of thinking persists. Here is what I know about God, to whom they refer. God endowed women with Souls which are infused with Wisdom, and a Mind and Body keyed towards language, community, and survival. Women know that there is a right time for everything: for loving, for weeping, for playing, for planting, and for deciding about when to be pregnant. The <u>God</u> they want you to pray to loves women too much to ever deny her basic health care or the ability to make her own choices. God is the originator of both our intellect and free will.

Mom Held Me

In the voting booth
Mom lifted me to reach
a lever, pull the curtain closed.
Held me, pointed to each tab
for her candidate...I voted for her.
Dark, secretive, strange this booth.
Mom whispered, ~*You have a duty.*
~*Vote in every single election.*
~*Women fought to Vote.*
~*You need to honor that fight.*
The fight for the right to Vote.

Too young to go to school,
I pulled the lever to exit.
Click clank the machine tallied.
Walking home she explained,
~*People used to say women*
  didn't need to Vote, women
  ought to think like their husbands.
~*Not true, you don't have to think*
  like your husband.

Dad was kind but authoritative
temper easily raised—not Mom.
Patient as a bulb waits to bloom,
loved him with a mind her own.
Always pregnant. Five children,
two miscarriages, two abortions,
failed condoms, failed diaphragms,
wild me in the middle of it all.

Fearful I was as fertile as Mom,
I popped The Pill my whole bleeding life.
Grateful to be a generation of
women with choice, angry
choice is being taken away.
So still...she's gone now,

but still...I Vote for her. I Vote for Mom.

Freedom

The righteous yell "No Abortion!"
thinking they have the corner
on morality, but do not think
about the obligation of
raising an unwanted child,
or watching a tiny life
blink out in pain and terror
when its diagnosis
of only hours to live comes true.

Do not consider
the rape victim, no matter how young,
or the mother terrified by the abuser
of her children as they cower
and whimper at his rage.

What happens to individual freedom
when the most private decision
is on public display?

What It Means to Be Pro-Life

She held a cardboard sign that read, "I'm Pro-life, Pro-women, Pro-science, Pro-Earth, Pro-children!"

When the woman standing next to her paused drumming, I approached and asked, "Can you tell me more about your sign?"

It was chilly at the intersection, and she stopped to rub her dripping nose with her glove and looked me straight in the eye.

"You think those people who call themselves Pro-lifers give a hoot about these embryos once they are living, breathing children who need things? They are the very same ones who call women, 'Lazy welfare moms!'

"What these kids need is a safe home, real food, love and attention! And they need to feel safe in school! Not be in a school where they are required to do shooter drills and hide in darkened rooms behind locked doors! Do you think it's logical that these so-called Pro-lifers are against gun controls? They think assault rifles are fine even though more kids are killed in schools than soldiers are dying! It's idiotic."

The wind whipped up the amber leaves at our feet and her declarations had clearly left her momentarily weakened. "Can you hold my sign for a moment?" she asked.

I took it and she pulled a handkerchief from her pocket and gave her nose a good blow. The group of protestors was starting to disperse and I invited her to coffee at the Adagio. She took back her sign stapled to a garden stake and followed me inside. We managed to find a booth and I ordered. As we waited, she resumed her explanations.

"The crisis with our climate is going to take the lives of many children, mostly poor kids. And do the pro-lifers care about that? They are so thick-headed they think that Jesus will just rapture them up to heaven."

At that point, she gave a sad little laugh and I noticed tears leaking from her cornflower blue eyes. She used a napkin to dab her eyes. "This climate thing has me freaked out. We didn't get no rain at all last summer! And it was so hot people were going to the movies just to get outta the heat. In all my years in Bellingham, I haven't seen anything like it! And the fires!"

Just then they brought our coffee and we sipped in silent reflection. She looked at me with those clear eyes surrounded by a radius of crinkles and asked, "What about you? What keeps you up at night?"

Road Rage

On the corner
by Planned Parenthood
three old white men
carry mass produced signs
'Pray to End Abortion'
Why not
Pray to End Rape
Pray to End War
Pray to End Cancer
Pray to End Racism
Pray to End Miscarriages
Pray to End Infertility
Pray to End Pollution
Pray to End Wildfires
Pray to End Flooding
Pray to End This Madness

Part 2

Lipstick

A gold tube of lipstick rests on her vanity table. I touch its smooth ridges as I peer into the mirror and feel transported several decades into the past. I sit straight-backed on the round ottoman—pinks and reds in a gingham pattern pulled tight over the seat and falling into stiff ruffles just above the floor. Everything is perfect, everything is just so. The seat demands an elegance I conform to. An elegance my grandmother had when she sat before this same vanity table applying that same gold tube of lipstick. I remember faint pink lipstick-smooches ringing the edge of a white coffee cup with scalloped edges. Her instant decaf granules in the green can. When I inhale deeply I can conjure up her image at the kitchen table—cup in manicured hand, fingers idly flipping through the San Mateo Daily Journal. Lips pursed, she completes the crossword while the news drones in the background and I watch from the distance.

A ring of pink encircles her Virginia Slims, lying abandoned in the coral ashtray on her patio. When the California weather turns chilly she moves to the garage. A bar stool next to a counter with space for her newspaper, her crossword, her novel; a cheap black ashtray; a cheap black radio—she perches here with long slim legs crossed. With one elbow propped on the counter, she's the epitome of a Vogue model circa 1960.

Her lipstick-coated smile is calm and graceful—never raucous—in the pile of photographs she's left behind. She's there with her husband, her three children—two girls, one boy. Her husband cracks jokes, makes faces, is exuberant with his hugs and love. She holds herself apart in some way and I'm reminded of a museum painting: You can look, but do not touch.

When her children are grown and her role as den mother to the Brownies and Scouts ends, she sits before her vanity and applies her lipstick in smooth, sure strokes. In sensible suit skirts she'll work as the Patrol

Sergeant's Secretary at the San Mateo County Sheriff's office for 18 years until she retires and receives a gold clock for her service. Like so much about this woman, what she does there is a mystery to me. I imagine uniformed men rushing about while my grandmother sits poised at a typewriter, calmly transcribing notes.

The gold tube descends into the abyss of her gray handbag. She carries it with her to her various appointments—the hairdresser once a week to freshen the red in her hair and enhance the wave of her short locks, lunch dates with friends, the Redwood City Library, the Stanford Shopping Center to browse the racks at Nordstrom. She refuses to drive; she refuses to get a driver's license. When my grandfather dies after 40 years of marriage she relies on rides from friends, family, and the city bus. I imagine her on the bus seat, back straight, eyes refusing contact as she looks through the windows. A smear of pink looks back at her.

In an old Kodachrome photo of her and my grandfather, the reds of her hair and the pinks of her lips pop out of the frame. As always, the effect is classy, not garish or cheap. Large glasses cover her eyes, but her painted lips move in a coy smirk as she turns to the camera. Her skirt is slightly raised, revealing a smooth, shapely leg. My grandfather, balanced above her on a ledge, leans down towards her with a mocking yet serious look on his face. "Wowsa," I imagine him thinking and saying. Those lips of hers both admit and defy the camera's voyeuristic peek into her life. She keeps her secrets well hidden behind the pink of her smiles.

She wipes the color off before bed, leaving her lips pale and colorless. She tucks her hair into a shower cap before scrubbing her face and applying cold cream. She smells of bedtime and bathwater. Somehow, she still manages to look elegant in her faded blue terrycloth robe. Her lips are cool as they kiss my cheek. Her daughter yearns for more warmth, more affection, perhaps just a more visible imprint of love from my grandmother. I feel it is there but not in the way she might expect. It's there in the smile lurking beneath her lips and in the shine behind her eyes. There are depths to her I understand more as I age, and I fear we are more alike than my mother might wish. I breathe a hot kiss on my mother's cheek to warm the pink one left behind.

My grandmother's image zooms into the computer screen as we adjust the picture on this video chat. Her hair is no longer red, her lips no longer pink. She will be gone in two weeks, though I'm due to be at her house in a month and five days. She is propped in bed against several stark-white pillows and morphine clouds her brilliant eyes. I know she's still there behind the pain, though. I can see it as I hold up my two-month-old baby for her to see. Her first and only great-grandchild. She's tearing up and I'm trying not to. Instead, I'll talk of how she'll get to hold him when I visit next month for Christmas. In our hearts we know the truth.

The vanity table is empty when I sit on the ottoman for the last time. I sit poised and straight-backed as I look in the mirror. My lips, colored only by the youth of my late twenties, tremble slightly. I think of my memories: how hard it was to keep her on the phone until I asked questions about the book she was currently reading, how she sent a Christmas ornament to me every year since birth until she learned my mother was keeping them "safe" until I settled down, then she mailed them to me directly, the way she hugged in such an awkward yet fierce way, her laugh, the way she chewed salad.

Sitting at her vanity table—such a sacred place—I wonder how many moments she sat here, alone, or otherwise. Did she ever slouch in grief over the grain of her wood table? Did her hands ever falter as they applied color to her lips, painting away whatever emotion she wanted to repress? Like me, did she ever wonder how she was supposed to do all of this and fit herself into the image of a mother everyone expected even if she didn't quite fit? If I could color my lips, I would. If only to feel that somehow I was keeping her legacy alive—that by painting myself I was covering myself in the woman I longed to know better.

Seventeen Bits of Bad Advice

1. Don't get so angry; it ruins your pretty face.
2. We hear you best when you use a conversational tone; no need to yell.
3. Dressing like that is an invitation to perverts.
4. If a boy starts kissing you and you kiss back, you'll get what's coming to you.
5. If you hear screams, run in the opposite direction. Don't get involved.
6. If you sit like that, no one will ever want to marry you. Act like a lady!
7. Don't start crying just to get your own way.
8. If you hang out with those anti-war hippies, people will think you're a communist.
9. Eat a sandwich before he takes you out so you can eat daintily.
10. In a town like this, everything you do will follow you. Do you want to ruin your reputation forever?
11. No one ever gives you anything "for free." Mark my words, their gifts will have strings attached.
12. Men like to feel sexy and proficient. No harm in faking an orgasm.
13. Family members are more important than any friends. Family alone will see you through hard times.
14. If you want to keep your job, don't make waves or ask so many questions.
15. Don't complain about your husband. If you don't want him, I'm sure some other woman would be glad to take him off your hands.
16. Pretend you don't know the answers; no one likes a smartass.
17. Who do you think you are? No one cares about your spiritual insights or beliefs. Get real!

Idaho

Once I lived in your garden.
A potato, I grew easily.
No watering, no weeding.
Green leaves, purple flowers.
Bursting with nutrients.

Buried just below frost,
you dug me that winter.
That winter I sustained you.
No consideration for the heart,
you slathered me with butter,
ate me skin and all.

Natural Phenomenon

Today started out sunny, but this afternoon the sky is clouding up. Several days have passed without lightning activity. The smell of rain wafts through the open window. To the west, sheets of virga, rain that evaporates before hitting the ground, cross Camas Prairie. Jack points out the virga and says there's another natural phenomenon that is visible to the naked eye. He crosses his arms over his chest in a stance of authority. "It's called prana: sparkling particles of life force."

Still acting a bit standoffish from last night when I turned down his sexual advances, he takes my hand and leads me out on the catwalk. I go willingly, happy that he wants to mend fences. In the distance, I see the storm gathering energy. Anvil clouds spread wide on updrafts. Maybe we'll get some action later, after all.

Jack leads me to the railing on the west side of the tower, facing the prairie. "Now look without looking at the air directly in front of you."

I relax my eyes. As I do so, tiny dots of light begin to dart around like sperm under a microscope. "Are you sure it's not just tired eyes? I mean, it's been a glary day."

"It's life force, you know, God," he says. "Remember when we climbed Gunsight?"

"Sure." I recall sitting on the pinnacle, my legs hanging over the rocky edge of the 7,000-foot peak. Sparkles swirled all around. The curve of earth at the horizon was obvious and blew our minds. The sound of universal *om* was nearly deafening.

"Everything's saturated with life," Jack says, narrowing his eyes. "And if we watch closely, we can see it."

I linger, watching the distant storm clouds piling up through the misty life force. Jack returns to the cabin. Soon I hear the familiar jingle of our *Green Acres* show on the battery-powered radio. Back inside, I gather my crocheting and take a seat in the green chair. Last bits of sunlight break through the clouds, warming the cabin.

Jack sits on the bed, angled so he can watch the building storm. He announces that he's seen a few pink flickers. "Cloud-to-cloud lightning!"

"Record it in the strike log."

"Fuck the strike log," he says, taking out his pipe and his stash of weed.

"Right," I say, and we both laugh. "It's impossible to get them all down. I hate the strike log."

Soon Eva Gabor's character, Lisa Douglas, is chasing escaped pigs around the yard. One has gotten inside the farmhouse. Jack doubles over laughing. I shift in the chair, unbuttoning the top button of my cutoffs. I'm not sure why I'm feeling so uncomfortable. It's not my time of the month.

Although I've wanted a baby since I was sixteen, my cat may be the only child I'll raise this lifetime. She's curled up next to Jack right now, sound asleep. I recall the glowering looks she gave him when we first started sleeping together. A stray who showed up on the apartment house steps after I moved away from home at age eighteen. From the beginning, Jude slept curled against my belly beneath the bedcovers. When Jack moved in, she left my side and sat at the end of the bed, glaring at the intruder.

Lisa chases pigs around the kitchen. They squeal and Jude gets up and jumps on the counter, looking around the room for the source of the noise.

"It's just the radio," I say, catching a flash of light beyond her. "There's one!"

Jack nods and continues to listen. *Green Acres*, as usual, is a fiasco. The Douglas's finally corral the porkers and Oliver heads off to town to do some banking. It becomes hard for me to listen, since I feel a headache coming on. I recall having a murderous migraine before the miscarriage. People say miscarriages happen for a reason. Everyone seems to have a story about the one, two, or five miscarriages they had before delivering a full-term baby. The stories are usually relayed with cheer, as if God's plan to wash away a child in a flood of red is no big deal.

I should have gone to the doctor sooner, but I'd read in Adelle Davis's book, *Eat Right to Keep Fit*, that it isn't necessary during the first trimester. The nurse was surprised I hadn't been in, but thankfully she didn't scold me. Over the phone she told me to stay in bed until I saw the doctor on Monday. And, not to worry. *Right!*

The sun's down now. I put away my crocheting and get up to light the propane lamp. I heat water for tea. Maybe I lost the baby at three months because Jack was so angry at me for getting pregnant. He'd been adamant about not having children for six years. But then the IUD fell out; I was sure it was a sign.

"It's raining," I say, seeing a weak flash far off to the southeast. "See that one?"

Jack acknowledges the flash with a grumble. I understand his desire for freedom. I know that he believes when you're young, you have plenty of energy to do whatever you want. When you're older and your energy is lower, there's plenty of time to work. He believes in opposites. If everyone works during the day; we should work at night. If everyone works while young, we should work while old. So now we're working during the summer, saving money to live on during the winter. We'll move back to Spokane and live in the green house where I miscarried. We'll cross-country ski every day and sit by the popping wood-stove at night.

Just like that it's pouring rain outside. The distant cloud-to-cloud strikes peter out. I get up from the chair and note in the strike log the few I

48

recall. Lisa Douglas complains about farm living. She pleads with her husband to move back to New York City. For some reason, she reminds me of my mother.

Jack lights a pinch of weed, offering me a hit. I decline, getting up to make tea.

At the doctor's office, the nurses inserted a catheter to gather a clean urine specimen to test for life. I cried the whole time I laid on the table. The nurses said they were sorry. Their kindness was comforting, but I knew the baby was gone before the test came back.

After the D&C I needed bed rest. Jack let me know in no uncertain terms how he felt about waiting on me. He can be such a prick. Maybe he's right, he *won't* make a good father. It's been two and a half months since the miscarriage, and he's shown little sensitivity to my feelings. The doctor said to wait at least three months before getting pregnant again. I guess there's no harm in trying!

The lightning show, for what it was worth, is over. Jack turns off the transistor radio. We brush our teeth to the sound of rain pounding the shutters. Jack switches off the gas light. Outside, a blue glow surrounds the shutters and runs along the railings, dripping down the uprights, lighting up the night.

"Fucking-A!"

I follow him onto the picnic table where we sit side-by-side, mouths agape as every drop of water that runs along the shutter edges and down the rails glows blue. We sit cross-legged, shoulders touching, as if we're watching a rock concert, taking in the natural phenomenon, our minds completely blown.

"Saint Elmo's fire," Jack says. We watch the blue plasma trail along shutter edges, dripping streams of glowing rain onto the catwalk. The luminosity runs along the railings and down posts in rivulets, spattering and spraying off sharp edges, every droplet lighting the tower like Christmas.

Jack strikes a match on the seat of his cutoffs and tips the flame to his pipe. He puffs, and the scent of glowing weed fills the air. Laughing, he says, "Out of sight, man!"

"What causes the blue glow?" I say, breathing in the smoky air.

"We're in a charged field from the thunderstorm. It happens at sea, too, St. Elmo's fire surrounding masts and rigging and sharp edges."

"But what makes it glow?"

"Static electricity."

We watch until we're too tired to watch any longer. Then we strip and climb under the covers, tangling bare limbs together. We kiss a little, drifting off to the sound of blue rain sheeting off the shutters, streaming down to the ground, refreshing the forest all around.

100 Words About Three Wrinkles

Once, I took a palm reading class. I learned that when I rolled my left hand into a fist, the wrinkles that formed where my little finger connects to the palm represented my future children, three. This sounded like playground folklore.

I had an abortion at twenty-one, terrified of consequences my inability to stand up for my body, myself, might bring. Then, I married a man who didn't want children. We compromised at one. Our first try bled out in cramps and silence. At thirty-one, our beautiful daughter tangled into our heartstrings.

On reflection, maybe those three wrinkles held true.

Dissected

I

Once I dissected a frog
the skin slipping
from my fourteen-year-old fingers
as I fumbled to secure the pins,
blew aside hair tendrils
caught between my lips.
The skin was pork chop pink,
layered like flakes of ginger
sitting next to the sushi plate
my first date had yet to touch.
Make sure you use the correct tool,
my biology teacher coached.
I thought of repeating the phrase
as my date reached for his fork.

II

After the frog came the cat
and I shuddered to see the plastic
snuggling the cat's waiting hips.
But with the cut came the beauty
of liver nestled below diaphragm,
an advent calendar of surprises
awaiting each tender lift and cut.
We named the cat Fred,

my lab partner and I.
Sorting through the viscera
my lab partner looked up:
I love you, you know.
But I didn't know
and all I could smell
was the formaldehyde
wafting over my senses
as everything else went dark.

III

When they cut out the baby,
ripe from my womb,
I lay on a steel dissection table
watching blue gloves carry
a scalpel out of view.
I felt the pull, the tug from within.
A merciless elf tickled my
endometrium,
the smell of intestines drifted past.
Then the gloves returned to hold
that small, wriggling form:
We've got a healthy girl here.
I couldn't move, couldn't reach.
Like a flayed animal I remained
motionless.

What I Want Most In Life

Jack and I met and fell in love when we were juniors in high school. He was way more experienced than me sexually and soon had me down to my underwear, begging me to *do it*. He said I would like it. He said it was the in-thing to do. I said no. I wasn't ready to have *sex* with anyone. All Dad's illicit touching had me wary of intimacy. We held off until our senior year when I lost my virginity on the couch with its pattern of stagecoaches and horses galloping on. After that, there was no stopping us. We were like rabbits. By the time I turned nineteen and Jack twenty, we celebrated our love for each other with a woodsy hippie wedding, against our parent's wishes of course, at Riverside State Park.

Real life has a way of getting in the way. By the time I turned twenty-four, with a miscarriage under my belt, I developed fibroids. My mother had recommended a specialist and I booked an appointment. He said the fibroids were keeping me from getting pregnant and we'd need to do exploratory surgery. "Unless you are a gambler!" he said. I didn't understand him at first and asked two more times what he'd said. Finally, he said, "Are you willing to take a risk, forgo surgery and experiment with hormone treatments?"

"Yes," I'd said, and that's what I did. I was glad I didn't go under the knife, for a year later the endometriosis had dried up. The process was just as the doctor had explained it, except for the *no period* thing while nursing. The curse came back the month following Keri's natural birth. The doctor said it was wise that I'd chosen natural childbirth, since the cord had been wrapped around her neck. Drugs would have only stressed out her body further.

Once home from the hospital, Jack and I ventured tentatively forth as parents, learning how to diaper and burp, feed and bathe, soothe and entertain our baby. I read Dr. Spock and together, we learned to be parents, which came more naturally for me than it did Jack. He was resistant, repeating his mantra often, hazel eyes squinting. "There's no way in hell I'm taking care of anyone besides myself."

He refused to change diapers. And if it did become necessary, he gulped down a glass of wine first and often threw up afterwards. And "baby sitting" while I spent time with my friends, was out of the question. According to Jack, it was my job to take care of the home and of our child. When I leveled with him about my nagging loneliness, he shrugged his shoulders and said, "Just gut it out, Nancerella." So, I shoved my sadness down and carried on.

Then Jack, with my help, applied for a good paying job in Yakima. He got it and we moved away from Spokane. Our families begged for us to stay, but we needed the money. Soon, there was no one to share the long days with, as Jack was working full time. So I spent my days nursing, cleaning, unpacking, and playing with our new baby. I pushed Keri downtown in her stroller, walking to the YMCA to water aerobics, working on getting my figure back. After that class, I signed up for a pottery class and participated while Keri played with other babies in the nursery. Eventually, I struck up new friendships—the kid Jack worked with had a sweet wife, though she was much younger than me. The neighbor lady who came over when we first rolled into the town in our big moving truck, invited us over for Spam sandwiches, which we took her up on. She said to stop by anytime, but I wasn't interested. Then a real estate agent started showing me houses for sale. We did want to buy something, and I ended up riding around with her so frequently that she and I became friends, wary at first, then for a while, fast friends.

Though I found making friends in an orchard town tedious and living across state from my family with a new baby, lonely, Jack's new job brought home enough money to buy food and pay off our hospital bill. Now, we had medical insurance and Jack had vacation and sick leave. But we still owed a lot of money for all the doctor appointments and the hospital. Slowly, we were digging our way out of debt.

Before the move to Yakima, even with unemployment insurance, we were poorer than poor. Thank goodness for food stamps and my sister and mother buying us bags of groceries now and then. My stepdad could have helped, but he didn't return my phone calls. He was remarried and his new wife encouraged him to forget my brother and me. After all, we were only stepchildren, not real children. He took her advice.

Overnight in the hospital and the delivery had set us back $600, which in September of 1975, we didn't have. After we got back home from the hospital, I was soaking in the bathtub with my infant curled on my belly when the phone rang. I heard Jack say, "What are you going to do, take the baby back?" Then I heard him laughing and saying something about a payment plan. I laughed too, splashing warm water over Keri's bare skin. I recall saying in that baby voice new mothers use with their infants, "We don't have to send you back." Keri gave me a sweet little smile in return.

In some ways, I think having a child made me feel more separate, more alone, since most of my friends are childless. Before we moved, I would cry and cry while Jack was away at Manito Golf Course mowing greens. I was tired from sitting up at night nursing and too sad to call my mother, sister, or one of the girls from beauty school, which I had taken time off from in my seventh month of pregnancy. They wanted me to come back once I had the baby, but the idea of leaving my infant alone with a stranger for eight hours a day, scared me to death. I decided I would find a school in Yakima to finish my training. Now that we live here, I realize my cosmetology license will have to wait. My focus is on raising my daughter. Motherhood is a responsibility, and I want to be the best parent I can.

I take a seat on the front steps and watch my daughter toddle after the cat, Cloud, who dives into the tall grass beneath the tall poplar tree at the edge of the yard. Keri goes after her. Cloud pops up and bounds out of the grass, racing across the yard. Keri shrieks with laughter and I laugh too, feeling in the moment happier than I've been in a long time. I am so glad we persevered and brought a child into the world.

Multitasking on Multivitamins

You say become a mother or else. I say it is not so easy. Have you seen the pedestal they put over there? The one ten feet taller than me? You must have heard the expectations of the mother pedestal. In order to ride this ride you must be: emotionally stable, gentle, patient, a psychic who knows when their favorite shirt needs washing, loving, supportive, able to figure out how to hide nutritious vegetables in their dinner, empathetic, authoritative yet kind, a mother who doesn't forget the water bottle when taking her kid to mountain biking class, consistent, calm, respectful, able to spend hours doing an activity that bores you to tears but excites them to no end, humble, an excellent lullaby singer, encouraging, willing to clean the 500 dishes making waffles for dinner entails because it's their favorite, positive, selfless, sleep-deprived with a smile on your face, generous, empowering, the sort of person who remembers your kid's height and weight at the oral surgeon—roughly the size of two dog food bags or three?, sacrificial, a coach/guide/cheerleader, a planner, an advocate, protective, willing to give up the freedom to eat potato chips for dinner, a teacher, understanding, polite, a domestic goddess, and, above all, a woman who is able to do all of the things before her first cup of coffee. I would finish this piece, but…my kid needs his scrambled eggs. With whole wheat toast and fruit. Yes, there's a glass of milk. And yes, a multivitamin, too. Jeez, what kind of mother do you think I am?

No Instructions on Motherhood

I don't know how to do this
    no guidebook
        no manual
            no Dr. Spock advice column
coaches me through. I don't
have innate abilities,
no intuition
just a sapling struggling
to push through the dark,
unknown canopies.

I can remember being a kid
on a swing set so high
singing badly.
Then I was free
no one to say
    do this
        not that
            stay quiet
                obedient
                    still
I have people to help
with examples of mothers
kind and loving.
My own was, too.

Yet expectations spelled out
in invisible ink
wrote over the kindness, the love.
Conditions that stall
an easy give and take

Had I not fought for perfection
I would not fight against shame.
It's no surprise
I blame myself
for anything
      for everything.

I can't speak the same love language
as natural to you
as the air you breathe.

I only know
to sputter forward
careful of my words
     emotions
         sorry
            I'll do better next time.

Take Down & Escape

When he passes out from too many shots of Southern Comfort,
you try to quiet his snores. It's something you've perfected, pushing
against his back with the bottom of your feet until he goes over. Only
once did he wake long enough to roll back and bring an elbow down hard
into the softness of your belly. That night, it was you who groaned as you
turned away. During the day, he is proud of his grit and muscle tension,
being a former wrestler familiar with take down and escape. "Isolate this
one," he says and touches a fingertip to your backside. But you can't rouse
gluteus minimus, medius, nor maximus in a singular controlled fashion. As
he coaches, his fingers eventually find your softness. You say you are busy,
as you have been resting there on the big blue ship of a bed all evening
long reading Carlos Castaneda's *The Art of Dreaming*. But his coaxing
eventually becomes insistent, which you know will take a hard come
about to resist, so you agree to his idea that you will continue reading as
he investigates your hold.

He finds you so beautiful, so soft, so wet. You drop your book and
the bed sets sail for the fringes of reality. You know what Carlos means
when he talks about dreaming, as gliding through giant filaments of
bubbling nothingness feels similar. Hubby's wiry system cruises on,
pumping away while you hover above the bed, watching pieces of
yourself scatter: humerus, femur, ilium, costal. It's when he collapses,
sweaty and spent, that you snap back, giving him a hard shove, feeling
both relieved and saddened at the same time.

"Your marriage," the psychic says, "is nothing more than a
maintenance marriage." She continues, those blue eyes of hers startling,
"The round shapes beyond your body are there for you to explore.
Nothing to fear out there in the cosmos."

Back in the bedroom, you say, "Ours is a maintenance marriage."

He steadies himself, arms crossed, one hand on his chin pulling at his beard. Curly strands drop to his T-shirt. He says, "But I love you."

"Do you mean you want me, you need me, or you're horny?"

He's quiet, not the same quiet that you are soothed by when astral traveling, but a thoughtful quietness that seems to keep him focused, as does picking at his beard.

"Right now, I mean I'm horny." He stops the whisker thing and reaches for your breast. "Come on," he says. "You know you want it."

You recognize those flat eyes, knowing that the light hazel will darken to cartoon-spiral-gray after a few shots of Southern Comfort, and his rhythmic humping will have him sweating copiously above you, a ship sailing against the current. And all the while your boney parts will scatter at odd angles across the bed and you will feel a terrible lightness lapping at the edges of your consciousness, buffering you until he completes course or gives up ship.

An Endless Winter Season

I spent years   untouched   though I slept with a husband
    every night   It can't be explained   the empty numbness
a terrible loneliness felt only when not alone   sorrowful cracks
          spreading   through inexorable ice
         as we ignored   the sound of splintering
Paralyzing cold   all those years   one endless
    winter season
   curled on my side   in darkness   night after night
       each of us   on the   very edges
of the bed Deep grooves   warped   the mattress
         a wide flat expanse
        between us
   a growing distance   no longer traveled
lands no longer explored   The memory has frightened me   awake
though less often now
       Mostly in hotels rooms
      those barren white sheets
       then at the end of a startling dream
       I'm drifting away
   broken loose on a king-size ice floe
         broken & adrift

To Me Alone

We stood on the bluff above the quiet bay.
The sun, hugged by islands,
finally set on waters, alone.

I held romantic images of you
standing next to me, embracing me—
but as always, you ran away
left me standing alone
by the trees guarding meadow cliffs.

Staring hard into the orange orb
its reflection seemed a sharp knife
scoring the water, pointing to me,
to me alone.

       I felt its blade burn into my eyes.

Honoring Your Vows

Over a decade ago, I chose a road I never thought I'd take and—to steal a line from Robert Frost—it has made all the difference.

I moved out, leaving behind a marriage to a good man who did his best to love me. Left behind beloved in-laws; my first home (where I'd finally removed all that damn wallpaper); a six-year-old dog we'd raised from a pup (and named after my mom); mutual friends who were our life's tapestry.

Divorce most often begins with women, and we're highly aware of how it will disrupt communities—many we've spent years building.

You can make yourself crazy wondering why you're unhappy when this is the exact image of happiness.

You can try to conjure gratitude a thousand times by recounting your blessings and end up feeling nothing but shame.

It takes enormous strength to open yourself up to public scrutiny. People want reasons. Many must blame someone for divorce to make sense. They can't see how two good people could discover they are mismatched and not work on it indefinitely. There will be mean-spirited rumors. Lost friendships. Terrible sacrifices. You will be tested. Knowing this causes a fear that makes many stay, deny and pretend.

Some couples may hang on for years and years, healthy or not, until the only loving thing left to do is to just cut the rope. Let go and free fall into unpredictability. Within that undeniable sadness, you can sincerely wish each other well, then land on separate, unknown roads of self-discovery. And, if you're lucky, as I have been, you may get to see the man you once loved remarry a kind, happy woman.

Paradoxically, when you make the choice to divorce, honoring the vow to love someone for life can be exactly what you're doing.

After It Ends

An unlit candle rests interred in a nightstand drawer

The sun is too lethargic to lift the leaden blanket
Near the rain-wet wooden bench, a prayer wilts in an empty pot

You taste thick dust as gray as real estate wall color,
while a neighbor's door shuts and muffles laughter

Sometimes you mosaic shards of regret into a tabletop

Your throat is the Grand Coulee dam
Crying in the shower is comfort food

Pages flutter to the floor from the loose binding of a book
reread and reread

The phone is a boulder

You're an angel
but you're white diet cake with no berries or cream

You snapdragon in fall, blooming
battered and pale against the gales

but the hummingbird has migrated

The Last Haircut

You lift a t-shirt over your head
sit pale and bare-chested
while I stand behind the kitchen chair
plugging in the electric shaver

The decision is final
the bags and boxes are packed
Who will cut your hair after this
I don't know

The familiar whir fills the silent room
my hand smooths over your balding scalp
I shear the sides in the conventional style you like
No other way seems possible now
that smooth, dark locks have turned
to rough, short pepper

I adjust the blades subconsciously,
knowing so well the space around your ears
around your temples and across your neck
where a shaggy field now sprouts
Places I once kissed with tenderness
now distant lands, both familiar and foreign

Cut hair falls down your back to the floor
I brush it from you quietly, concentrating
on each slow, final movement

You say a quiet thank you
walk to the shower alone
as I sweep the kitchen floor
and empty what remains

Life Drawing

His ragged breath begged me to hold my own,
the artist sitting next to me sketching with charcoal,

holding his breath as he rounded the curve of bosom.
Like a friend—I joined his audible breathing,
figuring it would steady my hand, an unbroken line

contouring the full-figured model's derriere. A smear
of black to shadow her inner thigh, white charcoal high-

lighting the pink flesh of breast. The torturous breathing
to my left continued like waves crashing on shore. Areolas

the color of anjou pears, a splendorous neck and chin line.
His ragged breath begged me to hold my own,

contouring the full-figured model's derriere. A smear
of black, the room's dank musk, the sweet scent of oil paint.
A prone silhouette like distant rolling hills, waist and thighs

suggesting the Palouse and its plowed contoured furrows
following lazy hills, spring wheat as green as fresh limes.

Women Bleed

"Women are very close to death
in a way men aren't."

Diane di Prima

We bleed monthly, most our lives,
sluffing unattached remnants
of possibility.   We miscarry.
Moments of hope swing to despair,
or not.   Perhaps gratefulness.

We approach the specter of death
with each birth,
                              stand on the precipice
as one life becomes
two.

We are haunted by death
when men push countries to war,
it is us women left behind
          to mourn.

Set it Ablaze

Fire is sanctuary
An altar to burn
Tinder of tiny troubles
Kindling of unkindness
Regret, shame, and worries
Gathered like dry wood

Set it ablaze
Torch it white-hot
Radiant flash and crack
Sharp spark and snap
A fiery pyre

Let it flame
Let it swelter
Let it be

Devoured

Warm yourself
in flickers and reflections
in curling sultry smoke

And when it seems
Nothing is left but ash

Be the phoenix
When you rise

Slow Dancing Alone in the Shower

High again, wholly alone this late night
long hot shower in the dark, feeling
steamy heat like a sultry nightclub

Water drops like mirror ball light
gentle reflections on warming skin
time suspended in peaceful euphoria

Soft face tilted to a falling stream
sweet smile spreading as my body
slow dances in my own encircled arms

Swaying side-to-side with intimacy
embracing nakedness and freedom
blessings raining on a radiant temple

Music emerges from within—
this is the sole song to dance to,
loving myself like this

Weight Loss

Have you lost weight?
Have you been working out?

Yes, I have

shed the weight of wondering
where men I loved would go
when we were apart

stopped consuming a load of lies
carrying countless secrets
dropped pounds of shame

finally let go of those heavy
self-doubts gained so gradually
so steadily for years without notice

Yes, I've lost the weight of dragging
out painful necessary goodbyes
cut the rope tied to an anchor of fears

surrendered the burden of believing
I'd be good enough if I just tried harder
to be a more lovable version of me

finally, I have stripped off layers of insecurity
exposed my soul free and unfettered
exposed my body bare and beautiful

And, yes,
after the weight has lifted,
I have been working out

whether or not
I've lost anything at all

now that I am light as thin clouds
I spread wings across the sky

Pantoum for Happiness

An August afternoon, flowers flowing over the deck
After youngest-of-five, crowded, hand-me-down days,
After random roommates, an ex-husband, some lovers—
There's no one but me in a new home, all mine

After youngest-of-five, crowded, hand-me-down days
Finally shedding ill-fitting clothes discarded by others
There's no one but me in a new home, all mine
I shine with pride, or I curl up with fear

Finally shedding ill-fitting clothes discarded by others
Am I a child running, playful and naked, or a woman exposed?
I shine with pride, or I curl up with fear
And, in-between these extremes, there's happiness here

The Gift of Self-Acceptance

When I was a 20-year-old university student, attempting to adjust to the idea of adulthood and independence while also dealing with a pattern of BIG moods, I was able to talk regularly with a counselor, Mike.

I once told him in a moment of despair, "I just can't keep up with the rest of the world." How could I live a life where I was always running and couldn't breathe? Why couldn't I ever allow myself to just slow down without feeling like I had a fatal flaw? I probably added in all sincerity, "Mike, how am I going to survive?"

My body's natural pace has always been different from anyone I've ever met. I was born a tortoise surrounded by hares, but I never seemed capable of winning any race no matter how steadily I persisted.

Mike's tone was surprisingly light for the profound response that followed. "It's not that you can't keep up with the rest of the world," he said. "It's that you can't keep up with the United States. Other parts of the world don't race like this, and you'd fit right in."

As an adult, I now know exactly what he meant. First in remote areas of Yunnan Province, China, and then on Pemba Island, Tanzania, where I was the first American guest at La La Lodge in a fishing village. Both felt like coming home.

In Pemba, others noticed and talked about it. Like Mike said, I fit right in. Locals invited me to stay. When the chief of the traditional tribe jokingly proposed marriage in front of a few new friends, they burst out laughing when I strung together a few words I'd learned in Swahili to reply, "You beautiful/great. Thank you very much. No."

In *The Geography of Bliss*, author Eric Weiner says world journalists use the term "gone native" for those who stay. Someday that will be me. Weiner calls us "hedonic refugees," people who have "a moment of great clarity when they realize, beyond a doubt, that they were born in the wrong country." Mike's insight proved to be true.

In my life, the right person always seems to show up at the right time. It's been a blessing. Unlike other big transitions in life, like adolescence or middle age, there's no name for that stage from age 18 to 25, despite all the growth and change. Mike was the mentor I needed. It always seemed like he had just the right life experiences, perspective, and wisdom to share. There were other epiphanies along the way, but I didn't recognize their full impact or the positive effect he had on the trajectory of my life until much later.

The story began with a referral from a campus doctor to the psychiatric clinic with a sliding fee scale for help with depression. I started hopping on the city bus once a week, traveling on Mt. Baker Highway to the edge of town.

The first visit to the clinic was scary. Following the right bus route and schedule, finding my way into the small building, walking up to the check-in counter, waiting surrounded by strangers. The counselor called my name and walked me back to his office while skimming my file. I'd hoped for a woman, but here was a man in his 40s, with brown hair, a horseshoe mustache, and a kind and calming demeanor.

He told me to call him Mike. As he leafed through notes, he said matter-of-factly without looking up, "I see we have a lot in common. You're a rape victim and I'm a Vietnam vet." I looked up in confusion. This was another profound comment in hindsight.

Then, when we settled, and he began asking me questions in that first session, no words would come. Literally. He sat quietly, gazing out his large office window. It was up against a forest and Bellingham was misty that day. I could feel the silence growing uncomfortably into long minutes while I tried to think of something to say.

Finally, I followed his peaceful gaze and watched the rain. He said, "I'm fine with silence as long as you need it, even if it's the whole hour." I could tell he meant it. Intuitively, and much to my relief, he relaxed and matched my slow pace. My first subtle lesson in self-acceptance.

Soon, after adjusting to the routine, I began to look forward to the regular bus rides, and especially to seeing the driver on my route. He was another man in his 40s, tall and lanky, with red hair and a handlebar mustache. Maybe he showed up at the right time, too.

I swear, that driver knew every person who stepped onto his bus. He reacted to each one with enthusiastic recognition. Many were headed to the same clinic, but they weren't fortunate enough to be able to hide their different mental afflictions in public like I could. These passengers were the types of people strangers surreptitiously stare at, then quickly draw their attention from in awkward embarrassment. But not on this bus. The bus driver was a hero to me. It's such a good feeling when someone's happy to see you, especially when they know you well enough to have a sincere chat as you pass.

This man was a gift, and it wasn't just the greeting. It was as if each week a different "regular" would take the seat near the driver for genuine conversation—light or serious. For me, counting the ride back, it could sometimes feel like I'd had one therapy session and witnessed two more.

We never spoke much, but it was impossible to hide where I was going each Tuesday. He'd ask, "How ya doing this week?" in a knowing way that wasn't intrusive, and I'd smile and give an honest reply in a word or two. *Not bad. Rough one. Pretty good.*

One time the driver's little girl rode the bus chatting him up behind the driver's seat. That day, he had two tiny ponytails on the top of his head until after she got off at her stop. All of us regulars were smiling at each other. We sort of bonded over watching the driver we loved with his daughter, acknowledging the dearness of it all.

End

You stand, tall and straight, a cross
Against the horizon. You have come
To your limit. Looking, you realize
The emptiness.

Vaster than the blue shield
Above you, your eyes run out
Farther and farther until they pull out
Everything inside you—leave only
Your shell, and that is nothing
When you have poured yourself
Over the endless miles of eternity.

Publication Credits

"Natural Phenomena" & "What I Want Most in Life," were excerpted from *STRUCK: A Season on a Fire Lookout*, forthcoming.

"Take Down & Escape," was awarded the Portia Steele Memorial Award for Excellence in Poetry, (2006).

"The Last Haircut," was previously published in Jeopardy magazine, #59, (2023).

"Fireflies," "Rights Period," "At Sixteen," "WTF," "Chasity," "Mom Held Me," and "Road Rage," were previously published in *She Votes*, (2022).

About the Authors

Nancy Canyon, MFA, is an energy healer, visual artist, author, writing coach, and astrologer. Her creative work reflects her personal journey of recovery from childhood sexual abuse. She holds witness, both with words and in the art studio, encouraging others to express their deepest feelings. Nancy is widely published with a book of poetry, *Saltwater*, and *Celia's Heaven* (novel) and a memoir set in Idaho, "STRUCK: A Season on a Fire Lookout." For more, see www.nancycanyon.com

Amy Alice has been told 3M times she's too sensitive. This collection reflects her beliefs that vulnerability is courageous, obstacles make us stronger, and authentic voices are powerful. Amy has always lived a quietly subversive life with bouts of tiny-huge, passionate adventures. When she was 19 at a Girl Scout camp in Idaho, she drove 100 mph on a dirt road, drank a beer and played pool at the Fighting Creek Tavern, and made it back in time for Kumbaya. Amy is grateful for the inspirational women of Wildhaven Writers and their role in her growth over the last 10 years.

Courtney Kendall came of age in the summer heat of an Idaho thunderstorm. She stays grounded through the magic of morning coffee, the soft weight of her lap cat, and the promise of peanut butter toast. She is a word weaver, forest dweller, ocean seeker, mountain gazer, book devourer, and in her previous life was terrified of writing creatively.

Suzanne Harris is an educator, ukulele enthusiast, poet, and writer. Since retiring, Suzanne has been enthralled with reading, studying, and developing a more nuanced understanding of our country's history. Mountains are her refuge, old growth forests are her peace-makers, and she loves to play in the North Cascades with her dog, Rizzoli. Her first book of poetry, *Sparks Along the Warp*, is forthcoming. She once drove through Idaho, but did not stop.

Rose McClean is a feminist and a forest worshipper. She believes peace on Earth will only be possible when the scale of power tips in favor of the Divine Feminine. She lives a solitary life with her twenty-year-old cat, Isis. Her bucket list includes: growing Idaho potatoes, learning to yodel, and swimming with a whale shark.

Leslie Wharton grew up as a feminist. Her mother took her to hear Gloria Steinem speak and brought her to Seneca Falls. This collection reminds her of the book, *Our Bodies, Our Selves*. She cherishes the friendship of her writer friends in Bellingham and wrote the poem *Idaho*, while working in her garden. You can read more of her poetry in her chapbook, *She Votes*. She is the co-author of the book *Phoenix Rising: Stories of Remarkable Women Walking Through Fire*. Find her work online at Wharton Studio Works.

Acknowledgements

Wildhaven Writers come together monthly to write and celebrate life. A big thank you goes to the following members for contributing to *Women's Bodies, Women's Words:*

Nancy Canyon for bravely leading the group over the past ten years, through a pandemic, and over many months compiling and editing this book.

Suzanne Harris for typing and retyping poems and essays, moving text about and shifting poems around, and for arranging the poems and essays in an excellent order that borders on superb.

Contributors and editors Nancy Canyon, Suzanne Harris, Courtney Kendal, Amy Alice, Leslie Wharton, and Rose McClean—good job!

Nancy Canyon, publisher at CanyonWriter Press, Ron Pattern & Nancy Canyon for cover design, Nancy Canyon for her painting, "Purple Bloom."

Thanks also to Paul Hanson at Village Books for his generous support of our writing group and Kelli Russell Agodon for her wonderful words summing up so articulately, our mission for writing this book.

www.ingramcontent.com/pod-product-compliance
Lightning Source LLC
Chambersburg PA
CBHW052117020426
42335CB00021B/2798